Nursing & Health Survival Guide

Portfolios and Reflective Practice

Sue Lillyman and
Pauline Merrix

T0033792

First published 2012 by Pearson Education Limited

Published 2014 by Routledge
2 Park Square, Milton Park, Abingdon, Oxon OX14 4RN
711 Third Avenue, New York, NY 10017, USA

Routledge is an imprint of the Taylor & Francis Group, an informa business

ISBN 13: 978-0-273-76066-5 (hbk)

British Library Cataloguing-in-Publication Data
A catalogue record for this book is available from the British Library

Library of Congress Cataloging-in-Publication Data
Lillyman, Sue.
  Portfolios and reflective practice / Sue Lillyman and Pauline Merrix.
    p. ; cm. -- (Nursing & health survival guide)
  Includes bibliographical references.
  ISBN 978-0-273-76066-5
  I. Merrix, Pauline. II. Title. III. Series: Nursing & health survival guides.
  [DNLM: 1. Career Mobility. 2. Nursing Staff--education. 3. Job
Application. 4. Professional Competence. WY 16.1]

610.4306'9--dc23
                                                              2012002316

Typeset in 8/9.5pt Helvetica by 35

Printed in the UK by Severn, Gloucester on responsibly sourced paper

contents

Reflection and reflective practice are words that are often used within nursing and health care education and practice. Reflection and reflective practice are processes that you as a student and professional practitioner need to be familiar with during your training and throughout your career.

This book has been designed as a quick reference to assist you in identifying how you can develop reflective skills from practice and how you can then use these for essays, portfolios and following registration for continuing professional development.

This book is not designed to replace more comprehensive textbooks on the subject of reflection but to act as a quick guide for you to use while you are in clinical practice. The book provides examples of some reflective models that you can use and some uses for reflection and processes that will help you develop reflective skills and become a reflective practitioner. It includes how to write your portfolio and curriculum vitae and describes the clinical supervision process.

Reflection is an active process and does not just happen. It does take some work on the part of the student/practitioner. This guide, however, will help you through that process.

Reflection

■ WHY DO YOU NEED TO REFLECT?

- Professional body requirements
- for the Knowledge and Skills Framework (KSF)
- course requirements
- self-development.

Professional body requirements

The Nursing and Midwifery Council (NMC) requires all nurses and midwives to maintain and develop their practice throughout their career. The *Prep Handbook* (Post-registration Education and Practice), produced by the NMC, provides an outline of what it expects from each nurse and midwife. These requirements include

- Keeping up to date with new developments.
- Thinking and reflecting for yourself.
- Demonstrating that you are keeping up to date and developing practice.
- Providing a high standard of practice and care.

To do this, you are required, after you register, to work as a nurse/midwife for a minimum of 450 hours over 3 years and to have completed at least 35 hours of learning activity relevant to your practice within that same 3-year period. The NMC also requires that you maintain a personal professional profile. For this reason, reflection is important and when recorded can demonstrate that learning and development are continuing throughout your career.

Other professional bodies will also identify their specific professional requirements for each practitioner.

Knowledge and Skills Framework (KSF)

As well as the NMC, the NHS has produced the Knowledge and Skills Framework for all staff working within the NHS. Through this framework, all practitioners are required to identify that they have met the standards in order to deliver quality services to patients. This framework is about the application of your knowledge and skills into your practice and will be followed up in development review and your personal development plan.

Course requirements

All nursing, midwifery and health care professionals' courses will include some assignments that are reflective in nature. These will help you in developing those reflective skills for applying theory to your practice and prepare you to become a lifelong learner throughout your future career.

Self-development

As health care professionals there is a need to develop within practice, whether it is to become an expert practitioner within a specific speciality, develop and gain promotion or keep up to date with changes within the NHS.

All this reflection is expressive and is aimed at enhancing professional practice.

■ WHAT IS REFLECTION?

Reflection is a process that has been used through nursing, midwifery and other allied professional health education and practice for many decades. It is a process through which the individual can learn from, for and through their practice.

It is usually
- local and related to your actual clinical work
- generated by you as the practitioner
- owned by you as a practitioner.

Reflection can help you to
- relate theory to practice
- learn through practice
- develop theory from your practice
- justify your practice
- identify your values in relation to your practice
- celebrate your practice
- identify the need for change within your practice.

Reflection-on-practice

Reflection-on-practice was a term developed by Donald Schön who suggests that it is looking back at an experience and then learning from it. Most of the reflection that you are about to complete for your essays and portfolios will include reflection-on-action, i.e. reflecting on events after they have occurred. Through this you might want to change some of your practice, justify your practice and even celebrate that practice.

Reflection-in-practice

Reflection-in-practice is another term developed by Donald Schön and refers to the reflection that happens while you are practising. You do not always have the luxury of taking time out to think about what you are doing, especially in an emergency situation, however, you can draw on past experience and bring those experiences/action plans into play. You do not work as a nurse, midwife or health care professional on 'automatic pilot'. Practice involves thinking about what you are doing and reflecting on past experience. It is not always a formal written event but can be thought through at the time of the event.

Anticipatory reflection

Anticipatory reflection was identified by Van Manen as a way of action planning before the event occurs. Reflection is a cyclical event as you can see from the models examined later. Sometimes you start to evaluate, analyse and plan an experience that you are anticipating before you get there, for example your first day on a new ward or clinical area. You think about what you might do, how you might react, how you felt on your last placement; this is the analysis and action plan before the experience. Then you have that experience and reflect on the experience afterwards to see if it has worked out as you planned and maybe you decide it has or that you need to rethink this for the next time.

Reflective practice

■ WHAT IS REFLECTIVE PRACTICE?

Reflective practice is the way in which you can conduct and learn from your practice. It is how you develop throughout your training and career. A reflective practitioner questions their practice, develops practice and *learns* from that practice.

■ WHAT IS A REFLECTIVE PRACTITIONER?

A reflective practitioner is someone who is constantly learning from and for their practice. They are practitioners who have developed critical thinking skills and are able to make decisions about their practice based on solid and defensible knowledge.

A reflective practitioner is

- self-aware of their practice and behaviour
- ever changing and developing practice through problem-solving behaviour
- able to analyse and evaluate their practice
- a critical thinker who incorporates theory and evidence into practice
- able to use ethical decision making
- able to justify their practice through evidence-based practice
- able to hold reflective conversations with others.

■ WHAT IS CRITICAL THINKING?

Critical thinking is central to reflection and becoming a reflective practitioner. It assists you in making those difficult decisions, justifying practice and identifying how you have arrived at your decisions based on a sound knowledge base.

Tools for reflection

There are a number of tools that can help you to reflect on your practice. These tools include

- critical incidents
- learning journals
- mind maps
- models of reflection
- critical friends.

■ CRITICAL INCIDENTS

Critical incidents were identified in 1954 primarily by John Flanagan, who worked as an aviation psychologist in the US Air Force. His particular interest was to review information in relation to effective and ineffective behaviours. Through observation, he was able to analyse incidents and produce critical behaviours for certain tasks. In 1984 Patricia Benner suggested that critical incidents could assist the development of expertise in nursing. She suggested that, by observing your practice, you can identify any effective or ineffective practice for the task you are undertaking.

Identifying a critical incident

Critical incidents happen all the time to all of us, but are unique experiences for each of us. For example, if this is the first time you have taken a manual blood pressure, it can be a critical incident in the way you learn from the process. Learning here comes in the form of the actual procedure, communicating with your patient, positioning your patient, record keeping, listening skills, etc. When you have been performing this task for many years and you have learnt the technique and perform the procedure as an expert, it is no longer a critical incident for you.

A critical incident can be
- an everyday experience
- something that is a new task/procedure
- something that went very well
- something that did not go to plan
- an experience that demonstrates theory learnt in class transferred into the workplace

- an experience through which you have learnt
- part of any aspect of care, including clinical procedural tasks, interpersonal or interactional situations.

They may not necessarily be major events even if the word 'critical' or 'incident' in health care makes us think they must be. However, try to think of them as 'learning events' instead. Although you can, and should, learn from these major events there are many times that you learn through your practice when things are going well. Learning in practice is a continuous process.

Writing a critical incident

Once you have identified an incident, you need to keep a record of it as a reminder for when you come to write it up as an essay or part of your portfolio. You can make a short note in your journal using the following headings. This should be recorded on no more than half an A5-sized notebook.

Incident number		Date	
Tick relevant box(es)			
Communication	☐	Service improvement	☐
Personal and people development	☐	Quality of care	☐
	☐	Equity and diversity	☐
Health, safety and security			
Factual brief description of the event			
Immediate learning points			

After you have recorded this you can refer to it at a later date in order to write a full reflection.

■ LEARNING JOURNALS

Learning journals, logs, diaries are all the same thing in this context. As part of a course, you might have been asked to maintain a log/diary/journal. These are private and confidential records of events that happen to you in practice. They are kept as a record that you can then draw on later to develop critical reflection for an essay or as part of your portfolio. You can use the critical incident layout offered as a guide.

You should not include any confidential information in your diary/journal/learning log such as

- patients' names
- colleagues' names
- ward or location information
- specific details that could identify the people involved.

What you should include in your journal/diary/log:

- summary of the events
- facts relating to the incident
- immediate learning points
- thoughts/feelings at the time.

Once you have started your journal/diary or log, you can use it to inform your practice by analysing why you felt this was a learning event/critical incident for you in the first place. You can use other formats, rather than just writing; these can be video diaries, audio recordings, photos, art, etc.

Example of journal entry

1st January 2012

Today I took my first manual blood pressure. The patient was a 65-year-old man who had come into the medical ward with shortness of breath. He appeared very frightened and anxious and had only been on the ward for half an hour. I took his observations with the help of my mentor. I felt nervous that I would not be able to hear the blood pressure and that I would get it wrong. I took it and my mentor checked it. I recorded the results and felt happy that all went well. I still need to practise a little more.

Here is the same incident using the critical incident sample format provided earlier.

Incident number: 24		Date: 1st January 2012	
Tick relevant box(es)			
Communication	☑	Service improvement	☑
Personal and people development	☑	Quality of care	☑
		Equity and diversity	☐
Health, safety and security	☐		
Factual brief description of the event			
First blood pressure. 65-yr-old male on medical ward with shortness of breath			
Immediate learning points			
Felt nervous but able to take first blood pressure; need some more practice			

These are the basis of the reflection and act as an aide memoire for your reflective essays or portfolio where you go on to evaluate and analyse the critical incident.

■ MIND MAPS

Mind maps are useful tools to include within your journal/ diary/log since they are a pictorial account of the event and the connections to that event. They help you to make connections and draw the links and relationships between the events that you have experienced.

Figure 1 An example of a mind map for reflection about patient with shortness of breath

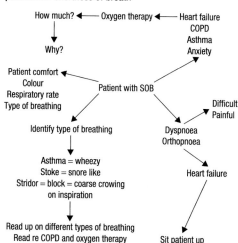

■ CRITICAL FRIENDS AND CONVERSATIONS

We need to be able to learn through our practice and one way is to talk with colleagues. Through using their experience and their helping you to understand your practice, you can start to develop your practice.

A critical friend can be
- another student
- a mentor
- a tutor
- another practitioner.

Critical conversations are
- constructive conversations
- helping you relate theory to practice
- an aid for developing theory from your practice
- a help for identifying learning
- supportive
- unusually with a peer (but can be with mentor)
- signposts for identifying action plans based on professional judgements.

They are not just chats with a friend with no outcome. They are conversations that lead us to think critically about practice, to apply new ways of thinking, to help us relate theory and, ultimately, to maintain a professional theory and evidence-based practice.

Models of reflection

There are many models that provide us with a framework for reflection. They are tools that, at the beginning, guide you through the process. It is good to use or base your reflection on a model but is not always necessary once you become used to writing reflections. Some of the more well-known models include Graham Gibbs' (1984) cyclical model of reflection, Christopher Johns' (2005) structured reflection and Borton's (1970) three questions. The choice is yours as to which one you can work with, like or find most appropriate for the incident you are recording. You can use all the models for different occasions or a mixture of them. Whichever model you use, the following elements need to be included:

- description
- analysis
- evaluation
- identification of learning
- action plan to return to description of new event.

■ GIBBS' MODEL OF REFLECTION

Gibbs' cyclical model (1988) is a useful one to start with and is set out in Figure 2.

Figure 2 Gibbs' model of reflection

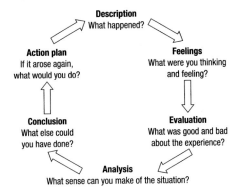

■ JOHNS' MODEL OF REFLECTION

Christopher Johns' model (1994) is also a very structured model that is divided into a number of cue questions.

The following cues are offered to help practitioners access, make sense of and learn through experience.

1 **Description**
   1.1 Write a description of the experience
   1.2 What are the key issues within this description that I need to pay attention to?
2 **Reflection**
   2.1 What was I trying to achieve?
   2.2 Why did I act as I did?
   2.3 What are the consequences of my actions?
        For the patient and family?
        For myself?
        For the people I work with?
   2.4 How did I feel about this experience when it was happening?
   2.5 How did the patient feel about it?
   2.6 How do I know how the patient felt about it?
3 **Influencing factors**
   3.1 What internal factors influenced my decision making and actions?
   3.2 What external factors influenced my decision making and actions?
   3.3 What sources of knowledge influenced, or should have influenced, my decision making and actions?
4 **Alternative strategies**
   4.1 Could I have dealt better with the situation?
   4.2 What other choices did I have?
   4.3 What would be the consequences of these other choices?

continued

5 Learning

5.1 How can I make sense of this experience in light of past experience and future practice?

5.2 How do I *now* feel about this experience?

5.3 Have I taken effective action to support myself and others as a result of this experience?

5.4 How has this experience changed my way of knowing in practice?

From: Carper, B. (1978) Fundamental patterns of knowing in nursing. *Advances in Nursing Science* 1, 13–23.

■ BORTON'S MODEL OF REFLECTION

Borton's model (1970) includes just three developmental questions that can be worked through

- What?
- So what?
- Now what?

This model appears to be very simple and, indeed, it can lead to superficial reflection if not unpicked at each stage. It can also help you to be more flexible and creative in your approach to reflection.

For example:

- 'What' This involves the descriptive and feeling stage that the other authors also note. You should include an outline of the event or experience to place the reflection in context.
- 'So what?' At this stage, you should consider the knowledge, skills and previous experience that you are basing your considerations on. You also need to explore

your decisions and actions and identify any other possible alternative approaches that you could have used.
- 'Now what?' This should include an action plan and a summary of your learning through the process.

■ PAAR MODEL OF REFLECTION

Another model is that of the Participatory and Appreciative Reflection (PAAR) model introduced by Ghaye et al (2008). This model very much relates to the positive aspects of your clinical work. It commences with reviewing what has gone well rather than what has gone wrong.

It consists of the following steps:
- Developing appreciations.
- Reframing experiences.
- Building collective wisdom.
- Achieving and moving forward.

■ OTHER MODELS OF REFLECTION

Here is a list of other people's models of reflection you might wish to look at:

1 Atkins and Murphy's (1994) reflective cycle.
2 Bolton's (2005) through the looking glass model.
3 Boyd and Fales' (1983) stages of reflection.
4 Goodman's (1984) levels of reflection.
5 Kolb's (1984) experiential learning cycle.
6 Mezirow's (1983) stages of reflection.
7 Rolf, Freshwater and Jasper's (2001) framework for reflexive practice.

The full list is much longer than this and you can find other models in the literature.

Learning through reflection

We learn for different reasons and in different ways:

- For our practice as a professional.
- From our practice as a professional.
- From observing others.
- From doing and learning through reflection.

■ FOR YOUR PRACTICE AS A PROFESSIONAL PRACTITIONER

Courses usually include some learning in relation to scientific/factual knowledge such as anatomy and physiology, politics and procedures that guide your practice and how to be a professional. These might come from formal lectures and reading. Many are facts that need to be learnt that can:

- guide you through your practice
- expand your knowledge
- help you to understand the theory in your practice
- help maintain your practice
- help to improve and/or change your practice.

■ FROM YOUR PRACTICE AS A PROFESSIONAL PRACTITIONER

You will learn much of what you do and how you do it as a practitioner by actually doing it. This is where reflection plays a major role. You can do the same thing 20 times and learn nothing or do it just once and learn a lot. This might be reflections as you are working (reflection-in-action) or after practice (reflection-on-action).

These can help you:

- translate the real world of practice
- generate theory from your practice
- to self-explore and develop.

■ FROM OBSERVING OTHERS

You can learn from your observing other people's practice, for example, observing what your mentor is doing. This can be in actions, attitude and/or behaviour.

■ FROM DOING AND LEARNING THROUGH REFLECTION

You can learn from trial and error, from using the reflective cycle and developing practice as you go along.

These can

- help you justify your practice
- make change happen
- turn change into improvement
- enhance your professional performance
- help you to develop and modify models of practice.

All your learning and practice should help you to gain the competencies identified by the NMC. These include knowledge, skills and attitudes you must acquire by the end of your initial training and maintain throughout your career.

These include

- professional values
- communication and interpersonal skills
- nursing practice and decision making
- leadership, management and team working.

Writing a piece of reflection

As stated earlier there are times when you are not completing a full essay but need to include a piece of reflection within a portfolio to demonstrate some learning. This might be as a result of a study day, to demonstrate a particular domain for the KSF, to demonstrate a particular competency for your training programme or to show that you have developed and achieved some continuing professional development for the NMC or other professional body. This reflection is much shorter than what you are required to write for an essay. Usually, one side of A4 is sufficient. You can use the following template to write the reflection.

■ FOR YOUR PORTFOLIO

- Short description of the event/experience encountered.
- An analysis and evaluation of the experience – draw on theories to inform your practice.
- What you could have done differently – this starts to relate that theory to your practice.
- What you have learnt through this exercise.
- What your action plan is for the future. Here you could include making sure it happens the same way again if it went well, further reading to gain more information, future course attendance or how you might adapt your practice to make improvements.

Writing a reflective essay

■ FORMAT OF THE REFLECTIVE ESSAY

These are usually written in the first person, but check with your tutor. The word count will depend on the requirements of the module.

Introduction

Summarise what you are including in your essay. Outline your content and identify the reflective model, if you are using one. If you say you are using a model, make sure this is evident (and make sure you follow it throughout the assignment).

Main text

This can be subtitled, especially if you are using a model of reflection. This helps to signpost the reader and makes sure the model is adhered to.

You should include a theoretical overview of the subject. Include general comments in relation to the area of the essay. You need to create a flow with an argument and reach a conclusion. There should be evidence of analysis and evaluation in this section and that all your work is supported with relevant literature.

Conclusion

Identify what the argument was and how you drew the conclusions you made.

References

Reference according to your university guidelines; these can usually be obtained from your library.

■ LEVELS OF WRITING

You can produce your essay at different levels. These include
- description
- analysis
- critical evaluation
- synthesis
- dissemination.

Description

This should be the first part of your essay after the introduction. It sets the scene and should only include enough information for you to make sense of the analysis. It forms the first part of your essay only.

Essays that remain descriptive throughout tend to gain low marks and often include little or no evidence of reading around the subject. This type of essay does not include any theory within the practice or state why it is relevant to the practice. It does not count as a piece of reflection but as an account of the event.

This descriptive stage should only form the first part of the reflective cycle, should be short and to the point and not form the whole essay.

Critical analysis

This usually follows the feeling part of the reflective cycle (see section on models). It is the main skill for reflective practice and your academic work and should form the largest part of your reflection when writing a reflective essay for degree- and diploma-level programmes. In this part, you need to provide evidence of what you are saying from the relevant literature. You need to undertake a detailed examination of the subject and ask questions about it. You need also to draw on theories that relate to the subject you are writing about. (For example, if your reflection is based on practice, you would need to include the NICE guidelines and pathways, what the current care is and where you read about it. You might include national statistics on the condition and therefore need to include where they came from.) You also need to think about alternative ways of doing that care and support that with the literature. This is referred to as 'critical analysis' where you do not accept everything at face value but can demonstrate rational and logical thinking to the essay. It should be logical, include an argument and arrive at a conclusion. This is a positive and constructive process not as the word may suggest a negative 'critical'. It is about identifying the strengths and positive aspects of the situation before identifying the weaknesses.

Evaluation

This is also part of the reflective cycle. When writing critical evaluation in your essay, you will gain a higher mark at diploma and degree level as it is considered a high-level skill. Evaluation is making a definite judgement about the topic you are discussing. You need to use a framework for an argument that is developed throughout the assignment. This argument should be strong and credible and persuade the reader to agree. It should include analysis of other authors' arguments, identify if there are alternative arguments, if the evidence is significant and/or if there are any assumptions made. It should assess the merit of any literature by judging how good, bad or useful it is. This section builds on the analysis to measure the value of something and create a strong and persuasive argument. You need to look beneath the surface of the issues.

Synthesis

This level of writing is usually for those at master's level and will involve being able to separate issues and then put them back together in a coherent manner. It involves separating the theory and generating new theory from that practice, bringing it back together using background information on a topic and then to reorganise it by topic rather than by source. To write at this level, you are usually an expert in the subject already. It also involves integrating new knowledge or fresh insight into a situation and then identifying any learning from it. It will involve moving practices on by changing ideas and making decisions based on past beliefs and values.

Dissemination

This is not usually required within reflective writing. This high-level skill involves becoming an expert in the subject and passing that information in a structured and informed coherent manner to others.

Some main points to remember when writing a reflective essay

- Use a clear logical structure.
- Base your analysis and evaluation on extensive reading around the subject.
- Include some independent thought.
- Do not include anything you have read without a reference.
- Do not waffle.
- Maintain confidentiality.
- Stay within legal and procedural guidelines.

Developing your portfolio

During your training and career you will be required to develop a portfolio of evidence that is used to assess your competence in practice. During any course, the format will be set by your university. Once you have qualified, it is an NMC/Health Practitioners Council as well as KSF requirement to continue and maintain a portfolio throughout your career. This portfolio for your continuing professional development (CPD) is not one profile but flexible so you can draw on different aspects for different occasions as identified in the following example.

REASON FOR PORTFOLIO	CONTENTS
For a job interview	Include information that demonstrates your ability to deliver what is included within the person specification and job description
To gain accreditation of prior learning for a course	To include the necessary information that demonstrates the worth of the course content and at the level required
For academic study	This is usually a set document and includes competencies that need to be achieved in order to pass the programme

continued

REASON FOR PORTFOLIO	CONTENTS
For your continuing professional development for the NMC, HPC or other professional body	This needs to demonstrate that you have updated your knowledge over the past 3 years and completed a set minimum amount of formal study (this can be completed through attendance at study days, courses or through private study that is evidenced)
KSF requirements for continuing professional development	This is a requirement by your employer if you work in the NHS. You require a portfolio that demonstrates your learning over the past year and it is used in your personal development plan. You should ensure that it includes all domains relevant to your role

There are a number of items that can help you identify that you have developed in your practice and these include

- certificates of courses attended
- certificates of study days (these need supporting with some reflection on learning, usually one side of A4)
- anything you have developed in practice such as
  - patient or carer leaflets
  - policies
  - guidelines
  - posters (photo is sufficient)

- any publications
- reading supported with a piece of reflection
- critical incidents that relate to your practice.

■ THE COMPLETE PORTFOLIO

It is useful to keep your portfolio in one place in order to draw out relevant information should you require it for any reason. You will not require all of it, but you will need to adapt it to suit the situation as noted in the example. The following information is a suggestion for the layout:

- Personal information: name, contact details, PIN number once qualified.
- General education: list in order and include certificates.
- Further education: list in order and include certificates.
- Higher education: list in order and include certificates.
- Professional qualifications: list in order and include certificates.
- Other professional developments: include your role in any professional groups, research, policy and procedure development, if you are a representative or lead in any area of care.
- Current employment: include an annotated job description and contract.
- Previous employment: include short summary of the role and job descriptions.
- Mandatory training attended: needs to be supported with the dates and a short summary of what you have learnt.
- Other study days: these are not assessed or mandatory. Need to include a short reflection of your learning, one side of A4.
- Additional employment: if you do extra work outside your current employment.

- Publications: include the reference and a copy of the article.
- Conferences: keep certificates and short reflection, one side of A4. If you presented, keep copy of programme and abstract and your presentation and/or photo of your poster.
- Personal appraisal: keep a copy of your annual appraisal that you have completed with your manager.
- Action plan/goal setting: form your action plan from your personal one. Could include a SWOT analysis for future development.
- Additional evidence: could include critical incidents, learning journal, photos that demonstrate something you have achieved.

Writing your CV

When you are going to an interview you will need to take your portfolio. As noted earlier, this needs to reflect the job description and person specification. It should not be a general portfolio that people have to read through to gain the information related to the job. You will also be required to produce a curriculum vitae when you apply. Here are some suggestions to include in a successful CV:

- Keep it concise: it should be to the point and contain only information relevant to the job being applied for. Usually, it should be no more than two sides of A4.
- Personal statement: it should contain how you think any experiences you have had connect with the job you are applying for.

- Do not leave gaps in work history: even if you think it is not relevant, you can make it so by including some of the transferable skills that the job gave you such as communication, leadership, team work, initiative, problem solving, flexibility/adaptability, motivation, interpersonal skills, numeracy and any IT knowledge.
- Up to date: your CV should be a developing document. If you maintain it as things happen you will not have to search around at the last minute to find items.
- Proof read: always make sure that both spelling and grammar are correct.
- Be honest: speaks for itself; although you need to sell yourself, tell only the truth.
- Include facts where possible: if you have some statements, make them, for example: 'Introducing a new system on the ward reduced bed occupancy by 10%.'
- Make it appealing to the eye: use bullet points and format it. Make sure it is easy to follow.

Read through all the application forms in their entirety as some people do not require CVs but a completed form only. Make sure you do as they have set out in their application procedure.

Clinical supervision

Another area in which reflection can be developed and supported is through clinical supervision. This was introduced into the NHS through the Department of Health's vision for the future document in 1993. The NHS defined it as:

Process of professional support and learning which enables individual practitioners to develop knowledge and competence, assume responsibility for their own practice and enhance consumer protection and safety of care in complex situations.

(National Health Service Management Executive 1993)

The NMC, through its Code of Conduct, and the Health Professionals Council endorse this as good practice. It also fulfils the government's governance agenda. Midwifery has a statutory supervisor of midwives who has statutory requirements under the Midwifery Rules.

■ WHAT CLINICAL SUPERVISION IS

- Voluntary
- non-prescriptive
- establishing its own ground rules
- supportive
- reflective.

■ WHAT CLINICAL SUPERVISION IS NOT

- Managerial control
- hierarchical in nature
- watching/supervising your work in practice
- part of your performance review/appraisal
- counselling
- a confessional
- a chat over a cuppa
- another hurdle to get over.

■ OUTCOMES OF CLINICAL SUPERVISION

- Identification of solutions to problems.
- Increased understanding of professional issues.
- Improvement in standards of patient care.
- Further development of your skills and knowledge.
- Enhancement of your understanding of your own practice.

■ FORMAT

There are several models for clinical supervision including

- one to one
- group
- networking.

The NHS trust that you work for will have a policy as to which approach it is using. The meeting, whichever approach is chosen, should involve reflecting on your practice in order to learn from that experience and improve your competence in practice. This can also be carried out in the form of action learning sets (see later).

■ PURPOSE AND BENEFITS OF CLINICAL SUPERVISION

- Main aim is to improve the quality of patient care.
- Safeguarding standards of care.
- Personal development of your professional expertise.
- Improvement in your performance.
- Staff investment on the part of your employer.

■ HOW IT IS CARRIED OUT

- Clinical supervision can be part of your preceptorship and/or mentorship when you first qualify or undertake a new post.

- Your supervisor should be someone you are comfortable to *share* experiences with.
- You should set the ground rules before starting (including confidentiality).
- It should involve some form of record keeping on your part. This can be a reflection on the process or the learning that can then be part of your portfolio.
- It should be a meeting that is usually held between you and your supervisor on a 4–6 weekly period and last between 1 to $1^1/_2$ hours.
- You should set the agenda with issues that you want to talk about.
- It should be confidential in nature and not identify or name any staff, patients or location.
- It should be held away from the clinical area so as to avoid interruptions.

■ SUPERVISORS

- It is advisable that you choose your own supervisors; however, they should be practitioners with experience in the subject in which you are working. They can be a peer or someone who is at a higher grade.
- Supervisors are often required to attend an in-house training programme in order to undertake supervision of others.

Action learning sets

Action learning sets are not an addition to clinical supervision but can be used as yet another approach to the process.

These are groups of people working at all levels of the organisation. In nursing, they were introduced by the RCN through its clinical leadership course in 2002. The aim of this approach is to do better things in the world and, through action learning, you can develop personally in the context of action on urgent and intractable social problems.

■ WHAT IS AN ACTION LEARNING SET?

- An action learning set is the framework that enables and supports action learning.
- It is voluntary.
- Usually consists of six to eight professionals.
- It is held away from the workplace.
- Regular meeting for set time.
- It includes a facilitator who guides the process.
- It is based on action from reflection.
- Three levels of development/learning include
  ○ about self
  ○ about issues
  ○ about the process of learning itself.

■ PRINCIPLES OF ACTION LEARNING SETS

- Provision of a situation in which practitioners feel safe to discuss practice.
- Gaining support from colleagues over any issues that the practitioner raises.
- Formulating their own action plans based on the discussions and challenges of their colleagues within the group.
- Reporting back on previous action plans.

- Participants are empathetic but do not provide advice; challenge and support the person with the issue and help their to develop their own action plan.
- Engaging in critical reflection to explore the issues raised within a social context.
- Feedback only given for clarification and to summarise issues; participant presenting the issue develops their own action plan.
- Avoidance of imposing values, opinions, giving advice, being judgemental, criticising or trivialising the person or their concerns.

■ BENEFITS OF ACTION LEARNING SETS

- Increase in personal confidence.
- Increase in self-awareness.
- Approach situations from a broader and more political perspective.
- Become more proactive than reactive.
- More reflective than emotional.
- Development of listening skills.
- Critical reflection forms an integral part of the process.

■ ROLE OF THE FACILITATOR

- Skilled practitioner.
- Commitment to ongoing education.
- Upholds the ground rules.
- Encourages group participation.
- Bounces ideas back for clarification.
- Helps group to highlight key issues.
- Helps group to expand vision.
- Questions to clarify, confirm and challenge the group.

■ TECHNIQUES FOR ACTION LEARNING SETS

These assist the group to question without giving advice, to probe for solutions and assist with the reflection. Groups may choose one technique or more that they feel comfortable with.

Some techniques might include
- DeBono's six thinking hats, six shoes or six medals
- Kipling's six honest serving men
- SWOT analysis
- forcefield analysis
- role set analysis
- perceptual positioning
- mind mapping
- appreciative inquiry
- brain storming
- concept analysis
- Z-technique
- circle of concern.

These are just some of the techniques available. There are other techniques that you might find are more helpful. The selection always depends on the group members' choice.

Summary

All of these processes, from the start of this book through to the end, are designed to help you as a practitioner to develop your competence and skill. They include techniques and are designed to assist you develop as a reflective practitioner. There are other techniques, processes, tools that you might find useful – have a look in the literature. We have presented

only the main ones here. You do not, of course, have to use all the methods and techniques listed. They are here for you to choose from.

Three important things to remember when using/writing for reflection

- Always maintain confidentiality.
- Be honest.
- Only work within legal and procedural guidelines and standards at all times.

References

Borton, T. (1970) *Reach, Touch and Teach*. Hutchinson: London.

Carper, B. (1978) Fundamental patterns of knowing in nursing. *Advances in Nursing Science* 1, 13–23.

Ghaye, T. and Lillyman, S. (2008) *Learning Journals and Critical Incidents* (2nd edn). Quay Books: Dinton.

Ghaye T., Melander-Wikman, A., Kisare, M., Chambers, P., Ulrika, B., Kostenius, C., Lillyman, S. (2008) Participatory and appreciative action and reflection (PAAR) democritizing reflective practices. *Reflective Practice* 9(4), 361–98.

Gibbs, G. (1988) *Learning by Doing: A Guide to Teaching and Learning Methods*. Further Education Unit, Oxford Brookes University Press: Oxford.

Johns, C. (1994) Nuances of reflection. *Journal of Clinical Nursing* 3, 71–5.

Lillyman, S. and Ghaye, T. (2007) *Effective Clinical Supervision: The Role of Reflection* (2nd edn). Quay Books: Dinton.

Useful web pages

Example of a reflective practice tool:
www.wipp.nhs.uk/tools_gpn/toolu4_eg_reflective.php

Example of Gibbs' reflective model:
**www.afpp.org.uk/filegrab/
gibbsmodelofreflection.pdf?ref=46**

Example of Johns' model of reflection:
**www.flyingstartengland.nhs.uk/reflective-practice/
reflectiveframeworks**

Example of Kolb's model:
www.businessballs.com/kolblearningstyles.htm

Nursing and Midwifery Council:
www.nmc-uk.org

Royal College of Nursing:
www.rcn.org.uk

Useful information in relation to reflective practice:
www.learningandteaching.info/learning/reflecti.htm